Sex: All about SEX

EVERYTHING you need to know about SEX

By Melanie Ng

THANK YOU!

Thank you for purchasing this book Sex: All About Sex. Enjoy and take advantage of what you will learn through this book. Thank You!

Table of Contents

Introduction

All about sex.

The contents of this book was accumulated from the answers collected in detailed interviews, which lasted anywhere between forty five minutes to two hours. The focal point of the questions was to learn more about optimal sexuality by learning about respondents' best sexual experiences, then tabulating their responses to come up with the most common factors. The study based their findings on a total of sixty nine participants, encompassing a diverse sampling of population. Those interviewed were men and women, diverse in age range, ethnic origin and sexual orientation; ages ranged from twenty three to eight two years of age.

Why sex is good for you?

Sex is a good exercise
Sex does a lot of stuff to your brain
Sex is also a form of beauty treatment.

The ten key components of phenomenal sexual experiences:

Being present, focused and embodied
Connection, alignment, merger, being in sync
Deep sexual and erotic intimacy
Extraordinary communication, heightened empathy
Authenticity, being genuine, uninhibited, transparency
Transcendence, bliss, peace, transformation, healing
Exploration, interpersonal risk-taking, fun
Vulnerability and surrender
Intense Physical Sensation and Orgasm
Lust, Desire, Chemistry, Attraction

7 Great Sex Positions to Spice Up Your Sex Life:

Lap Limbo
Sexy Sprinkler
The Lusty Lean
Mover and Shaker
The Wanton Wheelbarrow
The Sexual Seesaw
The Lusty Leg Lift

Why Sex is Good for You?

Except for contracting sexually transmitted diseases when you're excessively adventurous in this regard, yes, sex is definitely good for your health. I'm aware that it's a really old zombie topic (comes back to life again and again) and that most people have encountered this information before; but tell me, how many of you could still remember and enumerate ALL the benefits you'll get from sex? I doubt there will be at least one.

And so, in the spirit of pro-creation, pro-sex, and just for the heck of it, here's a quick (I wish) rundown of what YOU can get from sex:

Sex is a good exercise. Here's what you'll get for doing it frequently (masturbation is not counted).

Lower cholesterol – An aggressive and vigorous sex burns 200 calories. Do it every day and you'll have zero fat in your body, guaranteed.

Healthier heart – Not only will you lose weight, sex also guarantees a reduced risk of heart ailments.

Toned muscles - Muscular contractions during intercourse work the pelvis, thighs, buttocks, arms, neck, thorax, and PC muscles. Lazy sex will only get half of it. An improved PC muscle helps women relieve menstrual cramps.

Improved bones – more likely if you're into the acrobatic sex positions where you sometimes have to support your weight and your partner's. It's called weight lifting. Additionally, testosterone plays an important part here as well which will be explained later.

Increased blood flow – Sex helps increase the blood flow to your brain and to all other organs of your body. This leads to improved blood circulation which gives fresh oxygen supply to your organs and removes the waste products in your blood and organs.

Sex does a lot of stuff to your brain. Simply imagining it gets you through a lot of brain exercise. What more if you do it for real?

Reduced Stress – Good sex makes you release all that kept tension in your thoughts and just let go. Also, a study in 2002 reported that sexually active females whose partners don't use condom were less subject to depression compared to their counterparts whose partners did. They say that a hormone found in semen (prostaglandin) gets absorbed in her genital tract, thus modulating female hormones preventing the attack of depression.

Relaxed and Improved Sleep – Orgasms allows everyone to completely let go, hence a profound relaxation afterwards. Because of this people are able to surrender all distracting thoughts. Being able to stop thinking has helped many to overcome insomnia and have a better sleep.

Positive and calm disposition – Although not true for everyone, generally, sex makes you less irritable and gives you a positive attitude in life or about something. Sex is also capable of boosting your self-esteem.

Feel Younger – Aging folks always get that feeling. It could be, perhaps, attributed to the positive feeling associated with sex.

Relieves Pain – Sex is 10 times more effective than Valium. Immediately before orgasm, levels of the hormone oxytocin surge to five times their normal level. This in turn releases endorphins, which alleviate the pain of everything from headache to arthritis to even migraine.

Sex is also a form of beauty treatment.

Shiny hair and smooth skin – "Mane and Tail", which was first tested on horses, gives you shiny hair. Sex does better. Scientific tests found that when woman make love they produce amounts of estrogen, which make their hair shiny and skin smooth.

Healthier skin – Your skin gets smooth not only because of the estrogen but also because of the sweat. Especially during one sizzling hot and sweaty bout in bed, the sweat you produce cleanses the pores and makes your skin glow. Gentle, relaxed lovemaking also reduces your chances of suffering dermatitis, skin rashes and blemishes.

Improved Posture – Women who get regular sex not only get firmer tummy and buttocks, but also an improved posture.

Better Teeth – Seminal plasma contains zinc, calcium and other minerals shown to retard tooth decay. How then do you get it into your mouth? Girls, it's alright to get down and dirty. Additionally, torrid hot kisses encourage saliva to wash food from the teeth and lower the level of the acid that causes decay, preventing plaque build-up.

A healthy sex life also improves your sense of smell. Prolactin (a hormone produced after sex) stimulates the olfactory nerve, the center for smell, increasing smell perception. A lot of lovemaking can also unblock a stuffy nose.

Regular sexual activity boosts testosterone and estrogen levels in both men and women. Testosterone is what drives both men and women want to have sex, the more there is the more aggressive sex turns out. Besides boosting your libido testosterone fortifies bones and muscles. Some physicians suggest that testosterone keeps hearts healthy and good cholesterol high. Estrogen on the other hand keeps women's vaginal tissues more supple, skins smooth, and breasts soft and ample. It also reduces the pain of premenstrual syndrome.

Sex can also boost your immune system. People who have sex once or twice a week have been shown to have higher rates of immunoglobulin A, a known immune booster. Intimacy also makes human beings happy, healthy, and peaceful which dramatically improves the immune system and healing capability.

Your prostate will be happier when you have sex. That is because studies have seen a relationship between prostate cancer and the infrequency of ejaculation or the release of your man juice. When you're not able to release it, your prostate concentrates all the minerals of your seminal fluid up to 600 times. There's a possibility that carcinogens in your blood will also get concentrated along with it. So before everything's too late, just release it. Besides having sex, one effective way to combat the untoward effect of bad concentration in the prostate is a good old "Onanism". Onan your way to euphoria!!!

Perhaps, the best thing you could get from sex and the only thing you've been waiting to hear is; "Sex prolongs your life." A British study of 1,000 men found those who had at least two orgasms a week had half the death rate of their countrymen who indulge less than once a month. Just read the positive effects from the top up to here and you'll understand why.

One Round or More of Sex Bout

I think the best answer for this is: It depends on the couple on how they celebrate their sexual urges.

However, if you'll ask me what's better for me, then I will say that it's better to have one but long round than having more but short rounds.

What's the difference between long rounds and short rounds?

Well. In long rounds, say for example one hour round, the woman here will be enjoying much compared to the shorter rounds.

How would the woman enjoy this long and tiring round?
Okay… Sex is really tiring, whatever length of the activity. It just happens that in a long sex, both of the partners will enjoy exploring each body before engaging intercourse which is considered as the finale.

Let's not forget that male can ejaculate easily in just a short period of time, and the ejaculation marks the end of the sexual activity. While female can hardly reach orgasm.

In other words, male must consider that truth. He should do some ceremonies first to give time to the female partner to prepare herself, enjoy the pleasure of your touch, caress and kisses, and letting her reach the peak of the pleasure which everybody calls "Orgasm".

If say for example, you did your sex activity in an hour, to enjoy it, you will consume the 50 minutes on touches, caresses, kisses, even oral sex, and then the remaining 10 minutes will be for the real intercourse.

Secrets of Great Sex

Your friends have probably given you sex advice, you may have Goggled around for "hot tips," or maybe you even get your sex advice standing in line at the grocery store flipping through magazines. Spoiler alert: You can ignore most of what you've heard.

There is a lot of advice out there, and some good books about how to have better sex. Some people look for their pointers in pornography, or what they call their *"online sexual education."* But the truth is that most of the sex in movies, porn and in magazine articles is not actually great sex.

Maybe your friends told you a thing or two when you were out drinking, or maybe you picked up some tips in your last relationship. But as a Board Certified Sexologist and a PhD Certified Sex Therapist, I am here to tell you that what you think you know about having great sex is simply not the whole story.

Here are the 10 keys to great sex, and these apply to straight couples, gay couples, and young, old, married or living together.

Adrenaline, intense attraction, or the things they know how to do in bed; what is it about a sexual encounter that makes it so great? A group of researchers set out to answer this question and have recently released their findings in an innovative study published in the Canadian Journal of Human Sexuality (CJHS) entitled "The Components of Optimal Sexuality: A Portrait of 'Great Sex". They focused their attention on identifying specific characteristics that comprise 'great sex'. The investigation was conducted in the hopes of debunking sexual myths, and to offer a broader view based on a spectrum of sexuality. The outcome of such work offers a new way for people to view "human erotic potential and expand our understanding of what sex can be".

What Comprises Optimal Sex?

Sex is subjective. Many of the participants of the study put it this way, "no one can simply define 'great sex' for others". Yet their responses revealed a great deal of commonality, despite differences in lifestyles, ages and Sexual Orientation. Ultimately, the study illustrated that "there may be many routes to experience great sex, but the actual experience can be very similar across varying individuals".

Ten key components of phenomenal sexual experiences were identified during the course of research. Eight were deemed significant because they came up most often and were greatly emphasized by almost all respondents. The last two were characterized as insufficient in themselves to be necessary aspects of great sex, but were still considered by researchers as worthy of mention in the study.

Being present, focused and embodied

The state of feeling "totally absorbed in the moment", of being completely in tune with the sensations being experienced during great sex, was stated by interviewees most often and ahead of any other characteristic of an ideal sexual experience.

Another distinguishing aspect was the ability of respondents and their sexual partners to completely let themselves go during sex. They were unimpeded by distractions such as the mental 'running commentary' that many people have trouble shutting off.

Connection, alignment, merger, being in sync

Many of the respondents believed that a deep connection between two people, irrespective of the length of the relationship (hours to years), was a key component of optimal sexual union. Some described it as feeling synchronistic during intimate contact and a sense of merger, a "loss of personal boundaries, a distinct loss of ... self-awareness in the sense of separateness from the other". Others characterized it as a powerful energy and a sense of connectivity that kindles between two individuals.

Interestingly, with all this talk of merger and fusion, those who responded most passionately regarding this aspect of sex noted that the more grounded they were in themselves (with a strong sense of self), the more capable they were to let go with another. Additionally, they emphasized the need to set clear boundaries, accept themselves for who they are, and feel respected by their partner.

Deep sexual and erotic intimacy

The essence of this category is to imagine the undercurrent of intimacy two people develop long before they actually have Sex . The panel asserted a powerful connection between erotic intimacy and a sense of safety/security in a relationship. This affinity can be derived by a "deep mutual respect, caring, genuine acceptance and admiration". As it relates to this category of intimacy, practically everyone who participated in this study expressed the importance of a profound sense of trust between lovers.

Extraordinary communication, heightened empathy

The emphasis on communication doesn't stress individuals being technically skilled communicators as much as it underscores people's capacity to truly and freely share themselves. Participants articulated the importance of listening well and paying attention to verbal and non-verbal cues. They also reiterated the ability "to recognize (in a sexual capacity), even without being told told, what and when a particular kind of touch elicits a certain response in your partner and another does not." Non-verbal communication was seen as a vital component of transcendent sex. In order to successfully embody this element of sexuality interviewees stressed the responsibility of individuals to be emotionally mature enough to recognize their own needs and desires, in order to be able to convey them to their partners.

Authenticity, being genuine, uninhibited, transparency

One woman summed up these qualities as "sex where you can say anything and be anything". Authenticity in a sexual relationship involves individuals being entirely self-expressive, uninhibited and unself-conscious. With the results of this study continually building upon the importance of 'letting go' in relationships, the participants' data proved another important corollary; being so completely genuine with another human being has an incredibly powerful effect emotionally and sexually. 'Baring it all' was considered by many to be liberating and an important component of amazing sex. It also gave permission to their partners to be free to do the same.

Respondents attributed much of their success in coming to such a state of confidence and genuineness, to letting go of restrictive sexual myths and unrealistic expectations as it relates to eroticism.

Transcendence, bliss, peace, transformation, healing

The feelings of "bliss, peace, awe, ecstasy and soulfulness" were the signature characteristics of extraordinary sex. Some likened the experience to the transcendent feeling reached during meditation (such as found in Tantric Sex), while it reminded others of timelessness and expansiveness. Being able to trust your sexual partner enough to let yourself experience such intensity was seen as the fundamental basis of these factors.

Exploration, interpersonal risk-taking, fun

Participants of this study explained that great sex was a vehicle for them to discover themselves. By taking risks and pushing their own sexual boundaries, respondents felt a sense of adventure and personal growth, which in turn fuels further development and discovery. Many of them also agreed on the following, "What's sex without a little fun and laughter?"

Vulnerability and surrender

The ability to give oneself over to their partner was a distinguishing factor between regular and amazing sex. Being willing to let go and feel vulnerable were among the characteristics that allowed individuals to achieve this state of interpersonal sexual abandon. There is a way to tell whether you're truly surrendering to sex with your lover; as one interviewee put it, in unexceptional relationships, "There's always some maybe small but detectable barriers, some things held back. In great sex, I think those (for me) disappear".

Intense Physical Sensation and Orgasm

There were a range of opinions presented as to the role Orgasms play in great sex. Both men and women agreed that an orgasm was not necessary for a sexual experience to be considered exceptional. However, they noted that orgasms seemed to come naturally anyway when they were having 'great sex'. Some respondents also underscored the satisfaction they derived from a slow build up to pleasure.

Lust, Desire, Chemistry, Attraction

A striking conclusion drawn from the results of these interviews was the role that lust and desire played in amazing sex. They made it onto the 'Top Ten' list not because they were valuable in and of themselves, but rather because of their impact when they're mutually experienced. Whether individuals were drawn to one another through lust or attraction, their compelling chemistry influenced their perception of sex positively.

7 Great Sex Positions

The Lusty Leg Lift

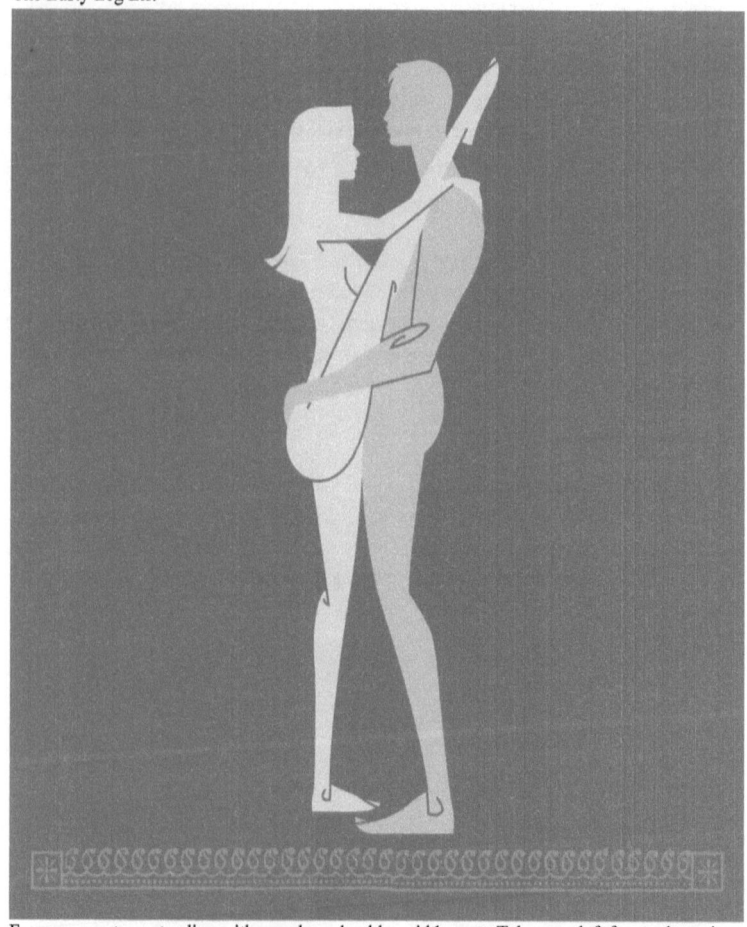

Face your partner, standing with your legs shoulder width apart. Take your left foot and turn it out to the side while keeping your right one facing forward. Have him widen his stance, with his legs about three feet apart, and then ask him to bend his knees ever-so-slightly. Wrap your arms around his neck and have him put his arms snugly around your lower back. Here's where it gets a little tricky: Pull your right leg up and place your right foot on his left shoulder, keeping your right knee bent. As he slowly enters you, ease into the vertical split by sliding your calf as far up his left shoulder as you comfortably can.

The Sexual Seesaw

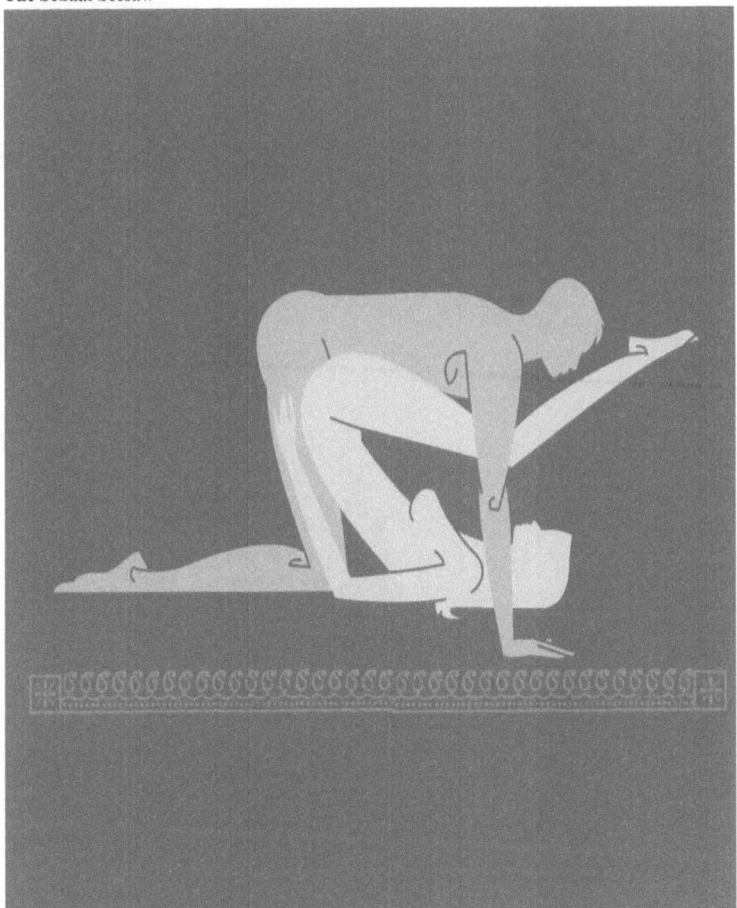

Lie on your back and lift your legs so they're over your ears and parallel to the floor. Your partner, kneeling in front of you, butts his knees up against your lower back, supporting you, and leans his torso against your thighs. (You can hold his legs to stay in this vixen-esque V-shape.)

The Wanton Wheelbarrow

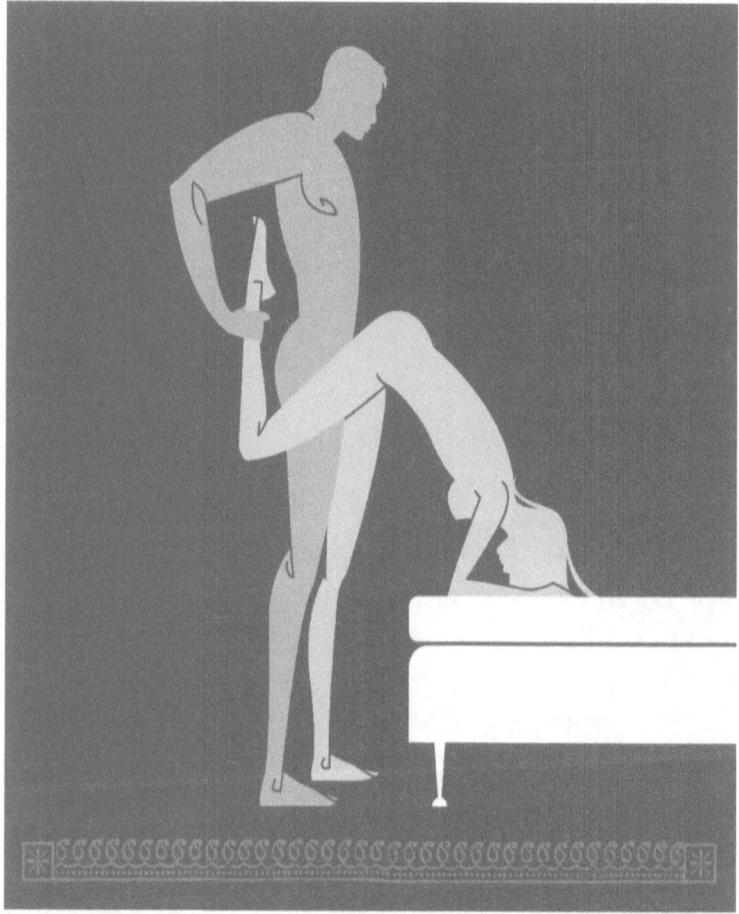

Start by standing and facing a bed or a chair. Bend over until your head and arms are resting on its surface. Have your man stand behind you and grab one of your ankles. Make sure to keep your knee slightly bent as you shift your weight to the leg that's still on the ground. Lifting your foot to rest near his hip, he should enter you from behind.

Mover and Shaker

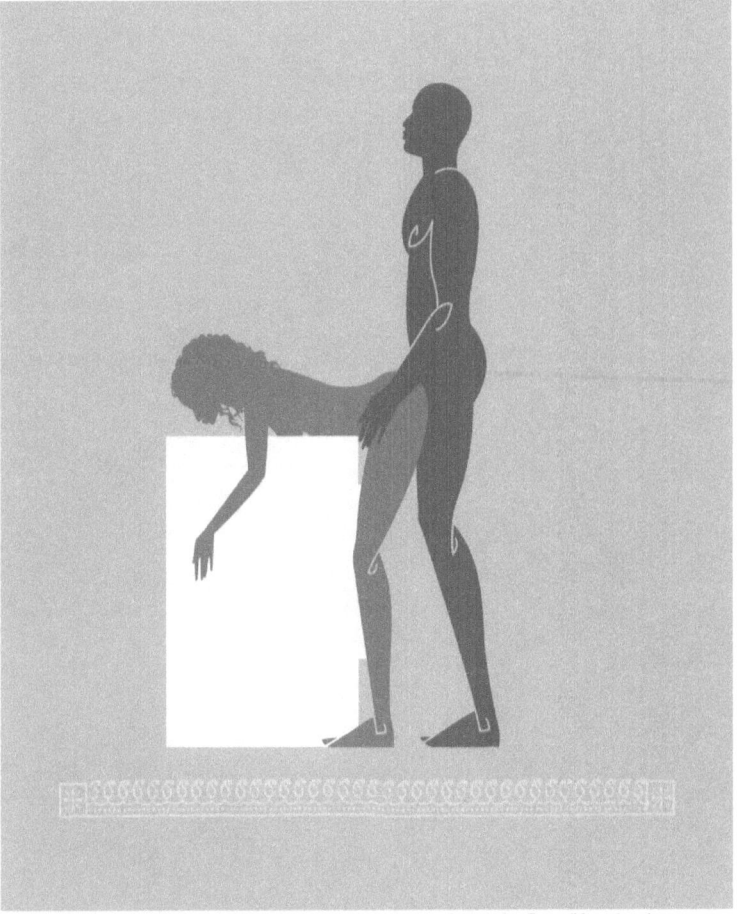

Lie facedown on top of a washing machine, with your feet flat on the floor (if you're short, try standing on a phone book). Have your guy stand facing your behind, between your legs. Once you're going at it, turn on the machine. Have him lean forward so that his thighs are pressed against you. The vibrations will rock through his entire body.

The Lusty Lean

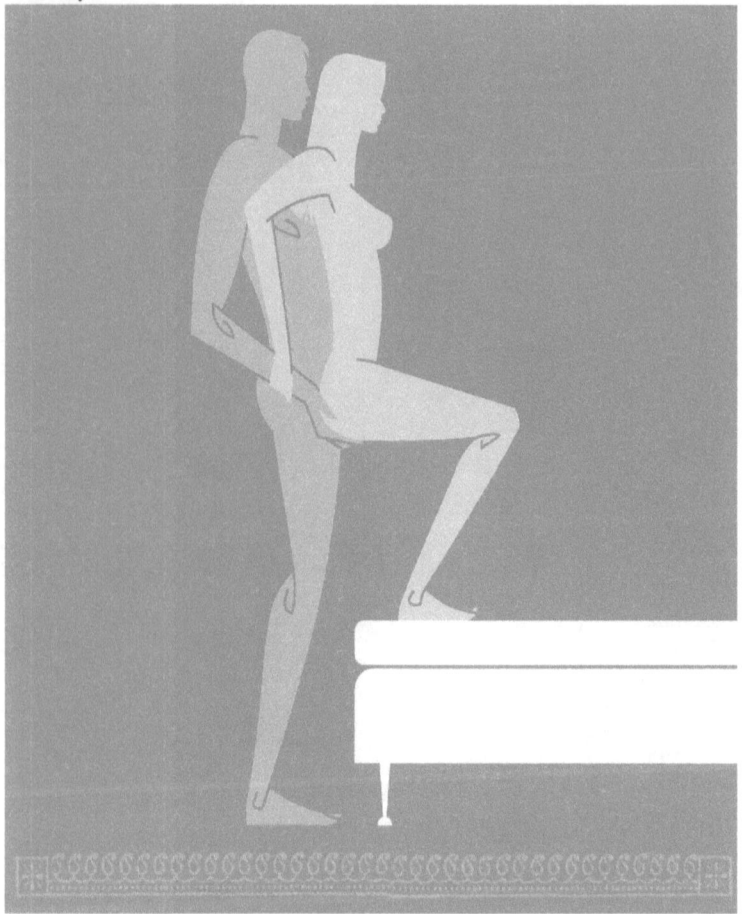

Your sweetie stands facing you as you squat on a bed or chair with your back to him. Lean on his chest as he steadies you by placing his hands under your rear. He then enters you from behind.

Sexy Sprinkler

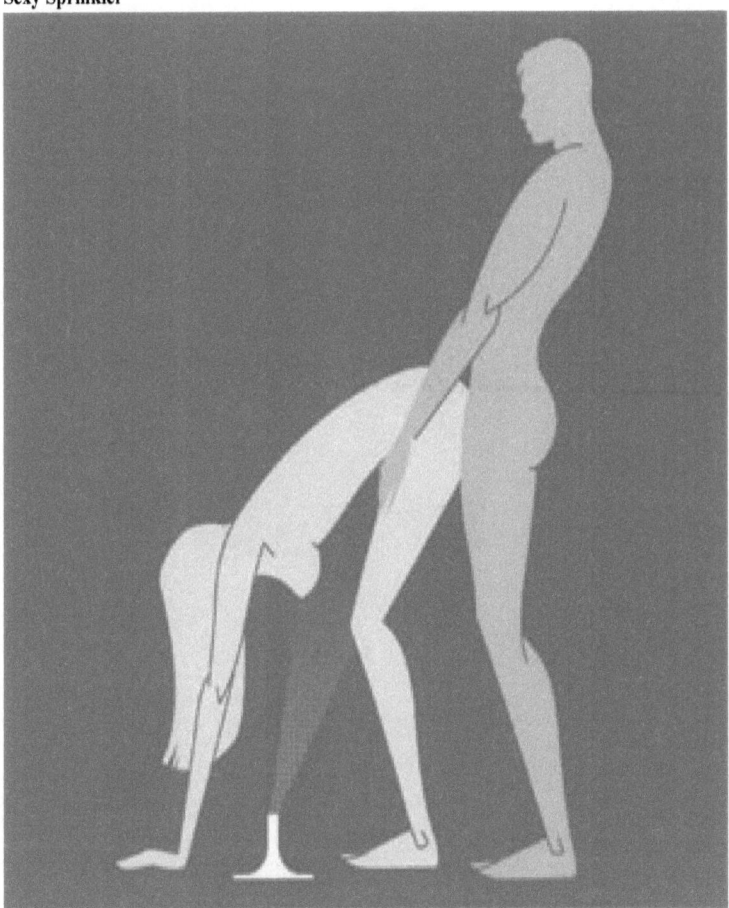

Save this position for a day (or night) when you two have the backyard to yourselves. Stand beside a soft-spraying sprinkler and bend over so the water hits your genitals. If you can't reach your hands to the ground, place them on your thighs or calves for support. Your partner should stand behind you and put his hands around your waist as he enters you.

Lap Limbo

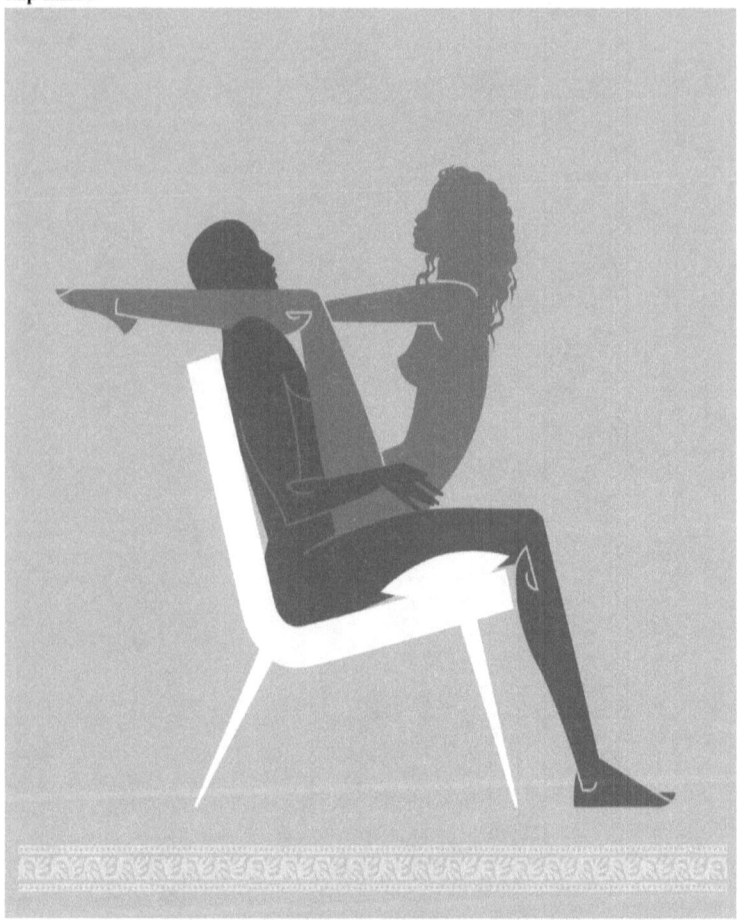

Your guy sits back in a roomy chair with a pillow placed under his knees to elevate them. Now you straddle him, lower yourself into the triangle of his lap, and lean back so you're resting against his raised thighs. Bend your knees and put your ankles over his shoulders so they rest on the back of the chair. He grasps your hips as he enters you, and you set the rocking in motion by pushing your feet against the top of the chair as he thrusts by pulling your hips toward him.

Breaking Sexual Ground

The study found that there was a lack of valid research regarding the nature of great sex, citing that experts in the field of Sexual Health actually have "minimal data on the farther reaches of human sexual potential". It also pointed out that other studies have a tendency to not take into account the broader spectrum of sexual function; they either take a more black and white approach, or focus too attention on treating dysfunction.

Final Thoughts

One of the most significant outcomes of this study was that the actual 'acts' performed during sex were deemed inconsequential when compared to the "mindset and intent of the person or couple engaged in these acts". These findings draw powerful conclusions about sex and healthy functioning, namely that individuals need not look outside of themselves to achieve great sex. Too great a focus on the physical mechanisms of sex will not be as fulfilling overall as the emotional, spiritual and psychological benefits of being present, embodied and vulnerable during sex. Additionally, the study encourages "comfort with self, personal and interpersonal exploration, revelation and acceptance". If an individual can achieve this level of growth, they are more apt to take risks both sexually and psychically, and can discover erotic attributes that they did not even know they possessed!

Great sex is private.

Some books will tell you that the only good orgasm is one where you stare at one another with open eyes while both of you climax at the same time. Really? I can't do it unless both my eyes are shut and I have a pillow over my face. Everyone is different.

Sometimes you might love to gaze into your partner's eyes. But there are going to be moments when the distraction of focusing on the other person takes away from the intensity of the experience for you. It is important to experience sex as it relates to you. Be selfish with your feelings, and take inventory of your reactions. This will allow you to go with the intensity and get lost in the experience. There is nothing sexier than a partner who is totally captured by you in bed.

Being ravished is wonderful, and being the one who ravishes is even better. But great sex happens in your own mind and in your own body. Don't ignore your partner because their pleasure will give you pleasure. But it is in your own private experience within that you will learn what you need in order to experience "great sex" moments.

There is a different between secrecy and privacy. Secrets are something kept separate and away from your partner. Private is a place inside where you cultivate and develop your sexual and erotic self. Your partner should encourage that part of you, because it adds excitement and juiciness to the sex for both of you.

If you have all five of these things; a plan, frequency, quiet, relaxation and privacy, you are having great sex, and congratulations! If you have a few, then you are lucky and you have some room for growth. If you aren't having good sex and you want more information, go to my website, drtammynelson.com, to find out more info or to buy my books. You deserve to have great sex and you deserve great advice. Don't settle. Great sex leads to a great relationship and a happy life.

Conclusion

Once again, I would like to THANK YOU for downloading this book.

I hope that I have been able to teach you all you want to know about sex through this book. I have tried to keep things simple as it should be.

Please don't hesitate to continue with your learning and go on to a more advanced program. Remember that having the right knowledge about sex is one of the key to a happy relationship.

THANK YOU VERY MUCH!

Please consider leaving a review for me at Amazon.com.